Ultimate Body-Building And Fitness

Contents

Body Building: Tips For Success

There are really two different ways of beginning a bodybuilding regime; the easy way and the hard way.

Which one of the two you choose for yourself will determine the extent to which you will stick to the regime and thereby prove a success. Since you have a choice obviously you will have to prepare a proper well etched out plan for yourself in order to select the right option. If you are like me (and like thousands of other smart people all over the world) you will no doubt choose to pursue the easy way, in which case you will have to start with a solid workout plan and get it all written down on paper.

Preparing a workout plan is in many ways comparable to the sort of New Year resolution planning we all tend to do. Of course most of us tend to give up the resolutions within a day or two, but here there is really no giving up.

Promises are hard to keep, simply because most of tend to make difficult promises. Most of us do not stick by the resolutions we make at the beginning of the year because our goals are not realistic. When we promise to quit smoking in the new year we ignore the fact that giving up smoking is a gradual process and needs time.

So the smart way to give up smoking would be to smoke about 4 cigarettes a day, then bring it down to 2 and so on. There is no point expecting to give up smoking just like that simply because we have promised to.

Similarly, when you plan your bodybuilding regime keep in mind that it needs a set of achievable goals to really work out. You wont turn into a Stallone in a month so don't intend to, give yourself a relaxed time limit of say 6 months for that. Also, remember when you are just beginning you will not have the kind of stamina a professional athlete or an experience bodybuilder will have so don't get disheartened if you can't keep up with Arnie (who has been practicing for 2 years now) on your first workout session itself. Don't make your gym session an ego tussle, you have nothing to prove anything to here. Take time relax and judge your progress astutely.

Ultimate Body-Building And Fitness

When you start your regime keep it to no more than 2 days in a week. Make sure you have at least 2 hours of time in your hand so that you don't have to hurry through the workout. Start with a few cardio exercises so as to charge your muscles up. Spend a bit of time on the treadmill or try some spinning, anything that will pump up your heart to about 80% of its usual capacity is a good choice. Even if you don't want to begin with the cardiovascular exercises make sure you do them after your exercise regime so as to help your body burn more fat.

<u>Body Building: When To Start And Stop</u>

Bodybuilding is a great way to sculpt your body into shape and lose those extra layers of fat. Training with weights can help you speed up your metabolism as well as tighten and define your muscles to give you that chiseled body. While that sounds easy, but don't be fooled into thinking that bodybuilding is a walk in the park. Bodybuilding does produce effects (there are thousands of people all over the world who would easily vouch for that fact) provided you stick to your regime, stay disciplined and work really hard.

As all of us who have tried to lose weight at some point of time know losing the fat your body has stored over time is not easy. It takes great devotion AND tremendous effort to finally bid it goodbye. This process itself can take a long time, as a result most people who take up bodybuilding often lose their patience midway and give it up altogether. It's not easy to keep working hard without seeing any effect of all your hard work on your body. But obviously the body takes time to react and it won't be prompt in responding just because we want it to. Staying with the regime requires tremendous willpower, a certain amount of faith and the knowledge regarding when to stop the exercising.

One of the very first things to learn in bodybuilding is when to stop. Most bodybuilding neophytes tend to keep working out till they almost collapse with exhaustion. Now, while pushing yourself is a good thing overdoing it is certainly not. Everything happens in its own good time, so no matter how hard you train right on the first day it is unlikely that you will see the effects of that training immediately. Also, intense exercises right at the beginning of the training can cause you to end up badly hurt.

Remember, to keep your exercise program interesting you must ensure that its fun, or else you will not return to it everyday and start avoiding it by some means or the other. Often heavy exercising can leave you feeling fatigued and hoping for a break. Under such circumstances do yourself a favor and take a quick break. Don't worry; some time off will have nothing but positive effects on your body. It will use the time you spend away from the weights to recover its strength and start building new muscles, thereby ensuring that your return to the weights will be in a far better form. But that's not all a break from exercising will also leave you feeling emotionally relaxed and at ease.

Ultimate Body-Building And Fitness

If you have just started bodybuilding you are probably yet to learn that that your body profits the most during the days when you stay idle at home instead of pumping the irons. This is because all the hard exercising can leave your body feeling tremendously fatigued. The short time off acts as a sort of 'recovery time' during which the muscles you crave for are actually created.

Muscle mass does not increase during your workout regime since muscles are too occupied working then. Instead, it expands in the days that follow your workout.

Thus, for maximum benefit and total muscle building increase the time you spend away from the gym and just relax, you won't regret the results.

Body Building: Time Management

You might have begun your bodybuilding regime but do you have a bodybuilding plan? Well, technically such a plan should include more than just lifting a few very heavy irons, gulping down some kelp and getting a tan to look macho. Like everything else the first rule in bodybuilding too is to get a plan and getting it down in black and white. The second rule, is to stick to this plan that you jot down and try and accomplish every detail it covers as closely as you possibly can.

One of the most important parts of your bodybuilding plan should be the amount of time you devote to exercising everyday, and how you manage to squeeze in that regime between your other chores. In time management we refer to immovable activities (that is the activities you simply HAVE to do during the prescribed hours) as 'Big Rocks'. So activities like say picking up your daughter from school or cooking a lunch or a violin class is all Big Rocks since you have to do them at the time when you have to.

So the first step to creating a bodybuilding plan is marking our all such big rocks in your daily agenda.

Once those are well marked simply select the time between them and squeeze in your exercise regime into them.

Now that was easy, wasn't it? Well it isn't the plan itself but sticking to the plan that is the tough part really. Try and be where you are expected to be according to your plan at all times. Don't be late, and don't spend extra time on anything, even the gym.

This brings us to the second part of that profound advice: DO NOT spend time unnecessarily, admiring your sculpted body in front of the mirror, or swaggering around on the dance floor showing off your newly chiseled body. Its true, you do look cool doing all of those but you'd look a lot better if you redeemed the time you are wasting in this manner and making use of it at the gym instead.

It's not easy staying motivated and distractions are rampant, like in every other field of life. To stay on the track therefore read books or listen to CD's regarding motivation, time-management,

success and competition. It's unbelievable, the kind of effect these have been known to have on people.

To upgrade and improve your bodybuilding plan stay tuned to the Internet. Filter what you read, because the majority of stuff you read online is bound to be written by seriously stupid, desperate wannabe's vying for attention. But not all of the stuff on the net is written by Moose. Keep searching the sites until you find a few which are actually helpful. Get your name included in their newsletter lists and read up the books they recommend you to. There is really no end to the extent such information can help you out. So look up the net and improve your plan today!

Body Building: Clothes

Most of us tend to be ambivalent about the kind of clothes we are going to be wearing during our bodybuilding exercise regime. While the puritans in the field emphasize that the regime itself is what is significant and not the apparel in which it is practiced, most others have come to feel differently.

All forms of exercises cause a lot of perspiration. While exercising for bodybuilding we work with a lot of weights, which causes our body to sweat profusely. To ensure that the sticky clamminess does not come in our way while exercising, we must wear clothes which can easily absorb this excess moisture and keep us dry at all times. Given its easy absorbing powers cotton is really the best fabric for all sorts of exercise wear.

It doesn't matter what kind of clothes you are ultimately wearing be it a T-shirt or a tank-top or even a fleece shirt, as long as its cotton you know you are on safe grounds. Pair up these with workout pants and you are all set for your exercise program. Bodybuilders, of both sexes, seem to be particularly partial towards tank tops.

Sportswear manufacturers have claimed it to be the hottest selling clothing item amongst bodybuilders. Tank tops come in a variety of colors, are generally cheap and therefore a good buy. It helps of course that tank tops allow a close view of the athletes pumped up muscles allowing them to get a good look of the kind of progress they are making. Bodybuilding has a lot to do with aesthetics, people who exercise do not just want a fit body they also want a beautiful body. A tank top allows them to flaunt this hot body. Some claim that there is nothing more motivating than being able to see your buffed up body in the mirror in front of you. A tank top makes such a view easily possible.

Despite all its plus points there are a few disadvantages of wearing a tank top. For starters clingy tank tops tend to keep your body wet and thereby miss out on the whole purpose of cotton wear. Clammy clothes can be a major issue while working out, hence a particularly tight tank top should be given a miss for a slightly loose one.

Secondly, a number of female bodybuilders are concerned about the amount of skin a tank top usually tends to show. Wear a tank only if you are comfortable in it, you don't want to be

concerned about what you are showing when you are concentrating on your exercise.

On the other hand, make sure you are not wearing something that is unnecessarily revealing, the gym is not a wet t-shirt contest and too much of skin can prove distracting for the others exercising around you.

Pair your tanks with a good pair of baggy track pants; these are roomy and therefore extremely comfortable.

Most athletes today are partial to a relaxed fit rather than the tight spandex fit that had been popular amongst previous bodybuilders. There is a range of such baggy gym pants available in the market today, they come in various attractive colors and are usually quite affordable.

Body Building: Understanding Anatomy

If you want to be an expert bodybuilder you will have to make an effort to understand your body's anatomy. In order to build your muscles adequately you will have to know exactly where each of them are located and how they might be developed successfully. This might sound easy but it is hardly a walk in the park, especially because of the often unpronounceable names of the muscles.

In order to know your muscles closely therefore locate a mirror and try and find each of the muscles on your body on your own. Let's begin with the neck. In your neck area there are two basic muscles you can concentrate on during your bodybuilding routine. These are the upper trapezius and the levator scapulae. The first one is the muscle that runs down from your nape to your shoulder.

The latter runs parallel to the initial cervical vertebrae in your neck.

The trapezius, fondly called the trap muscles climb down the nape of your neck and around the waist on both sides of the spine. On your shoulders you will find the deltoid muscles, also called the delts. On the front part of the shoulder is the anterior delt, on the side is the middle delt and on the back is the posterior delt. Just under the anterior delt you will find the rotator cuff muscles running straight out from the armpit area.

On the chest are your pectorals or pecs. On your arms you will find 2 different types of muscles, the bicep and the tricep. The triceps run down the side part of your arm from the shoulder till the elbow while the biceps run along the inside part. Both muscles are quite distinct on the forearms.

Your abdominal muscles or abs are located right on your stomach area.

On your legs you shall find the quadriceps muscles or the quads immediately in the front. The rest of the leg muscles are located on the back, on your calves i.e. the lower part of your legs. Yet another muscle, called the hamstring is located on your upper leg.

Yet other important groups of muscles include the glutes on your bum and the lats located on the upper part of your back. On your lower back you will also find the lower trap muscles.

Just like a sculptor ought to know both the material he/she is working on as well as the strokes he/she will be producing on it you, as a bodybuilder must also know your body (or your material) and your exercise regime (or your strokes) intricately. Knowledge regarding both of these essential factors is absolutely necessary for all bodybuilders. Unless you know your muscles like the back of your hand you will not be able to engage them and develop them adequately. Hence, begin your bodybuilding regime with a conscious effort to identify each of the important muscles on your body.

Concentrate on each or a group of them at a given time. Figure out how you want to shape your body in terms of the muscles you need to exercise and go about your workout accordingly.

Types Of Exercises

You may not be familiar with some of the terminology used in body building. Along the same line, you should know what certain exercises are and how to safely perform them. There are all sorts of exercises you can perform – so many, in fact, space prevents us from listing all of them. However, learning the basics can be a great help.   .

Dumbbell Bench Press

Sit on the edge of a flat bench with the dumbbells resting on your knees. In one smooth motion, roll onto your back and bring the dumbbells up to a position slightly outside and above your shoulders. Your palms should be facing forwards.

Bend your elbows at a ninety-degree angle with your upper arms parallel to the ground. Press the weights up over your chest in a triangular motion until they meet above the center line of your body. As you lift, concentrate on keeping the weights balanced and under control. Follow the same path downward.

Standing Military Press

For this exercise, you will use a barbell. Stand with your legs about shoulder width apart and lift the barbell to your chest. Lock your legs and hips and keep your elbows in slightly under the bar. Press the bar to arm's length over your head.

Lower the bell to your upper chest or your chin depending on which is more comfortable for you. This exercise can also be performed with dumbbells or seated on a weight bench.

Lying Tricep Push

Sit on a flat bench holding a curl bar with an overhand grip. Lie back so that the top of your head is even with the end of the weight bench. As you are lying back, extend your arms over your head so that the bar is directly over your eyes. Keep your elbows tight and your upper arms stationary throughout the exercise.

The biggest key to this exercise is keeping your upper arms in a fixed position. Slowly lower the bar until it almost touches your forehead. Press the bar back up in a slow, sweeping arc-like motion. At the finish, lock your elbows completely.

Side Lateral Dumbbell Raise

Stand upright with your feet shoulder width apart and your arms at your side. Hold a dumbbell in each hand with your palms turned toward your body. Keep your arms straight and lift the weights out and up to the sides until they are slightly higher than shoulder level. Then slowly lower them back down to your side again.

Keep your palms turned downward as you lift the dumbbells so that your shoulders rather than your biceps do the work. Make sure you are lifting the dumbbells up rather than swinging them up. Don't lean forward while doing this either or you risk injury to your back.

<u>Sample Meal Plans</u>

Choosing the right way to eat to build muscle can be a little overwhelming. But once you start eating the way you need to, it will become second nature to you. Following is a list of good foods for you to eat in each of the categories you need to concentrate on:

<u>Proteins:</u>

White meat chicken or turkey

Canned tuna

Canned salmon

Fresh Fish

Shellfish

Eggs

Tofu

Soy

Red meat like steak or roast

<u>Complex Carbohydrates:</u>

Oatmeal

Potatoes

Yams, Sweet potatoes, Acorn squash

Rice

Legumes

Corn

<u>Vegetables:</u>

All water based types.

Lettuce, Cabbage, Spinach

Asparagus

Bok Choy, Leeks

Tomatoes

Celery

Onions

Green Beans

Broccoli, Cauliflower, Radish

Zucchini Squash

Mushrooms

Carrots

Peas

Meal 1:

Vegetable omelet (3 egg whites, 1 whole egg, 1 cup veggies) You can also add some chicken or lean beef if you want.

Meal 2:

One cup yogurt or a protein shake

Meal 3:

6 oz Chicken

Small raw vegetable salad

1 bagel

Meal 4:

1 piece fruit

3-4 oz Chicken

Meal 5:

6 oz fish

1 - Cup grilled veggies

1 - Cup brown rice

<u>Sweet Dreams (Getting Enough Rest)</u>

Rest is one of the most overlooked parts of an exercise regimen, but the reality is it is actually a quite important principle. Sleep is one of your most valuable tools for growth that you can have in your body building arsenal.

Muscle adaptation and growth often occurs at night. During the suspended state of animation you are in, your body is doing exactly what you have been asking it to do during your workouts – build muscle.

Lack of sleep can have an intoxicating effect on your body. According to the Journal of Applied Sports Science, being awake for 24 hours has the same physical effect as a blood alcohol content of 0.096, which is above the legal driving limit in most states.

Working out in this state has its obvious downside. For starters, your lack of muscular coordination places you at a much higher risk for injury. Just as you'd never head to the gym after drinking a few beers at your local tavern, you should never work out after not sleeping the night before. You're better off waiting until the next day when your body has been given proper rest.

<u>Body Building For Her</u>

Many women are concerned with how their bodies look. Dieting and weight obsession are very real parts of life for many women. Body building and women really fit together well when you think about it. Focusing on healthy weight gain and muscle fitness makes a woman look and feel a lot better.

Body building is a lot more than just dieting and lifting weights. Much of the advice given in previous chapters can apply to both men and women. But women do need to change a few things when it comes to a workout plan that will work.

Some women have never considered body building as a sport because they are afraid that they will get big, bulky, and become masculine looking. Nothing could be further from the truth. A trim, solid body on a woman is extremely sexy and very healthy.

Women cannot naturally produce the amount of testosterone that men do, so it is impossible for women to increase their muscle size in the same ways that men do just by picking up a weight or two. Without artificial substances, women won't be able to get the same bulk as men do.

However, many of the same workout advice that we give to men apply to women as well: eat 5-6 small meals per day, drink plenty of water, and get lots of rest. The workouts are the same as well although some women may want to limit their reps initially until their strength is built up.

Many women struggle with excess fat and flabby muscle tone on their thighs and in their buttocks. Because women are naturally curvier than men, working these areas makes for a very flattering figure

Your Resources For Body Building

In this, the greatest information age ever, there are many, many places you can go to for answers to almost any question you have regarding body building. Seek out this information and learn as much as you can. This will make you a better body builder and a safer one at that!

To begin with, you need to subscribe to a couple of body building magazines. Some of the most popular include:

Flex

This magazine is considered the "bible" of hardcore body building. They do interviews with experts in the field and offer up some amazing advice for both the experienced as well as novice body builder.

Find them online at www.flexonline.com or subscribe to the paper edition for just $29.97 per year for 12 issues.

Nothing can really compare to personal advice and guidance. There are many gyms and fitness clubs that have local organizations dedicated to body building where you can get tips and train with others who share your passion. Ask around when you are in the gym, or network with others in social settings.

The Internet is another invaluable resource for body building information. In researching this book, this author depended on several of these websites for information. Here are a few you should really check out:

www.bodybuilder.com

This site is nothing less than amazing. You will find more information than you could have ever hoped for on this website including tips on nutrition, sample workout plans, and ways to prepare yourself for competition.

<u>Boost Your Metabolism Naturally</u>

When we are young, our metabolism is naturally high, but as we get older that just isn't the case. Do you remember the days when you could eat anything that you wanted at any time and never seem to gain a pound? Those days were great, and long gone. However there is hope. Of course we live in the age when we all want to find a quick and easy way out of everything. We want to find a magic pill that will change all of our lives, and the fact is there are thousands of them that claim to do just that.

These pills can be very dangerous and even deadly if they are not used properly. The good news is that you don't even need them. There are many solutions that you can easily use to boost your metabolism in a completely natural manner that will not cause more harm than good. The best thing that you can do is to exercise regularly and eat a balanced diet as is directed by the food guide pyramid.

Even if you have a medical condition that requires you to have a special diet, you can still boost your metabolism. Part of having a good metabolism is having good physical health and the other part is having good mental health. Personal fitness is very important in maintaining a high metabolism. This does not mean that you have to be skinny it just means that you have to be fit.

Drinking certain teas like green teas can also help you to detoxify your body which will also help boost your metabolism. Green tea has become very popular in the past few years as a means of doing this. Also, it is essential that I mention that a protein enriched diet will help you to build up your body's natural muscle mass as well. Adding certain vitamin supplements can also help you to boost your metabolism.

Vitamins like vitamin E, D, C, and B will be great for boosting your metabolism. If you don't like the idea of taking them in pill form you can find these vitamins in most fruits and vegetables that are in their most natural state or steamed. Green vegetables are great sources of natural vitamins and minerals that your body needs to stay fit and healthy. If you are dieting you should make sure that you are eating balanced meals. Getting healthy and boosting your metabolism should go hand in hand. Otherwise, you will only succeed in hurting yourself.

The South Beach Diet And Metabolism

The South Beach Diet claims that it is a scientifically proven program that is sure to help you achieve your goals and resolutions for losing weight safely. This diet will help you lose weight fast and improve your heart health at the same time. On average, most individuals lose between 8 and 13 pounds in the first two weeks when they start the south beach diet plan.

The South Beach Diet is completely different from the Atkins's Diet because it is neither low-carb nor low-fat. Instead, the diet teaches you to rely on the right carbs and the right fats. This process is made simple using a three phase process that begins with banishing your cravings and ends with installing a diet plan that is meant to last for life.

The real value in the South Beach Diet is the sound nutritional advice that you will receive. This diet retains the most important part of the Atkins's regimen, eating meat, while forgetting the philosophy that you can only eat low carb foods. Instead, you are encouraged to eat a well balanced diet for the remainder of your life. This sounds easy right?

The well balanced diet of the South Beach plan should be composed of plenty of fruit, vegetables and whole grains, nuts and healthy oils. Countless people from around the country continue to rave about the weight-loss success that they have experienced because of this diet. This program is easy to learn and put into practice, and is becoming one of the most popular forms of dieting around because of the success rate and dietary freedom involved.

Celebrities love the South Beach diet plan and swear by it. That is where much of the hullabaloo came from, but it doesn't mean that the diet doesn't work. The average person does find that this diet is one of the cheaper and easier ones to maintain since it requires balanced eating habits instead of deprivation. Perhaps that is why so many stay on this diet forever.

The South Beach diet offers a great deal of variety to what you can eat and makes it so that you can enjoy your meals without feeling hungry. This diet is easy to follow and is very worth the time invested in learning it. If you make it a long term part of your fitness program, you will notice that you have more energy and your metabolism will get the jump start that you need.

Using Food To Boost Your Metabolism

When most of us think about our metabolism it is mostly just in terms of losing weight. Our weight and our metabolism is what we use to define our bodies these days. The only problem with this is that we are also likely to forget that dieting does mean an absence of food, but the moderate intake of food. It is not healthy nor is it smart to take on all of those fad diets like the Atkins, South Beach or Zone diets that force you to completely give up certain foods because they only work for the length of the time that you are following that diet. If you do not continue that way all of the weight that you loose is only temporary.

Food is the key to boosting your metabolism and when it comes in its most natural forms, it can also be your best tool in maintaining a great weight for your body size and type. When I say natural forms I mean for example, when you eat vegetable and fruit it helps to eat them in the form that they naturally come in. if you eat fruit from a can, it is contained in syrup and sugars that will not be good for you so eating them raw is the best choice.

When you are eating vegetables it is best to eat them raw and steamed because it keeps all of the vitamins and minerals in them. You should also avoid processed foods and fried meats. Don't get me wrong fats are a necessary aspect of nutrition however saturated fats are not. The right balance of foods in a day can give your metabolism a boost that pills and fads can't.

It is best to eat at least three meals a day that are balanced with each food group as prescribed by the food guide pyramid and in between snacks as well. What people don't know is that it is ideal that you eat five small meals a day instead in order to get the most out of your metabolic system. The more foods that you intake in a day that are healthy the better to boost your metabolism.

It is not always easy for most of us to follow the food guide pyramid; however, it is still the best way to ensure that you get the most out of your efforts. Diet and exercise combined is the best way to boost your metabolism naturally, but if you can't do both walking and eating right is the way to go. There is no real excuse not to do both, but it was necessary to mention them.

The Harm Of Using Diet Pills

Diet pills, which are also commonly called appetite suppressants, have been prescribed by doctors since the 1950s. When they were first introduced to the public, the majority of diet pills contained amphetamine which is otherwise known as speed. This drug is highly addictive and doctors quickly realized that appetite suppressants that contained it would not prove to be the remarkable weight loss solution they were searching for.

As time went by, several other drugs such as fenfluramine and dexfenfluramine (which are more commonly known by their respective trade names Pondimin and Redux) came onto the market. Soon afterwards, doctors started combining a drug called phentermine with fenfluramine to form the now infamous fen-phen diet pill. Anyone who has paid attention in the last two decades will remember how badly that turned out.

Like all other drugs, weight loss drugs must be approved by the Food and Drug Administration (FDA) before doctors can legally prescribe them to their patients.
Not to mention that in addition to approving the drugs for human use, the FDA is also responsible for constantly monitoring the effects that such medications have on the health of the people who take them.

As a way to deal with the constant need for FDA approval and regulation, the active ingredient that is often used in many diet pills is not a drug anymore.

Instead, these products typically consist of naturally occurring herbs and are sold without a prescription over the counter. Perhaps the most popular herbal supplement used in diet pills is ephedra which is also found to cause major health problems. Green Tea and caffeine is also an extremely popular additive to most diet pills today. Hopefully we will learn that there is simply no safe diet pill on the market. We should all just stick to diet and exercise if we want to maintain a good weight.

Dieting To Boost Your Metabolism

Any person who is attempting to lose weight is always told to give some thought into researching all of the available weight loss diet plans before settling on one. Weight loss diet theories are located just about every where you look. The most popular one of the bunch appears to be the high protein and low carbohydrate plan that most dietary doctors use themselves and recommend to their patients. We all know that the key to losing weight lies in your metabolism.

The big emphasis that just about every sensible weight reducing diet plan should be healthy weight loss, not fast weight loss because many of the 'fast' diet plans are not safe or healthy. With this in mind, the best type of weight loss is a calorie reduced version of a healthy balanced diet. This diet should encompass foods from all the various food groups that are outlined in any food pyramid only in good proportion.

Many doctors and physicians who research weight loss are now starting to focus on how low carb foods can help people trying to lose weight. The low carbohydrate foods that are currently available are unlike all healthy snacks that have come before them. They are tasty, and because of their popularity they are inexpensive and can make an immediate difference in how you look and feel.

We all want to lose weight fast, preferably by eating our normal favorite foods. Unfortunately, successful weight loss means that you have to commit to a slow but steady weight loss process and a change of eating habits. The sooner you study which weight loss diet plans will work for you, the sooner you and all of your friends will see the new and improved you.

When it comes to time to choose the right weight loss plan that is based on food it is best to choose the diet plan that best corresponds to the types of foods that you already like to eat because this type of diet plan will be the easiest to stick to. Other than that, they all have their positives and negatives.

<u>Using Low Carb Diets To Boost Your Metabolism</u>

The low carb diet craze that is going on right now is an industry that is gaining momentum and demand every day and is showing no signs of slowing down. This is an amazing accomplishment for Dr. Atkins, whose book was immediately labeled potentially dangerous when it first hit the shelves years ago and again after he died. Now, every individual who considers himself overweight, and some others are hitting the supermarkets looking for the best high protein and low diet foods that they can find. The impact of low carb diets can be felt in just about every industry.

The thousands of success stories have people going to the gym at a record rate. They know that the Atkins and the South Beach Diet will help them lose weight, but they want to keep that weight off for as long as possible and so they automatically begin to get more active as well.

The major players in the grocery industry are now making even more space on their shelves in order to accommodate the low carb foods. Last, but not least, the low carb food manufacturers continued to thrive as their sales continue to improve at record levels. The low carb diets are even starting to have an effect on the menus at fast food restaurants. The wraps are actually very good.

No matter where you look, low carb foods are available for sale at reasonable prices. There is no simpler way to lose those unwanted pounds and keep them off. Low carb diets are here to stay. It's up to you about whether or not you should try the low carb diet, but if you do, it has never been easier than it is now.

You know that a diet plan is in demand if places like Subway and McDonald's is starting to accommodate it. Ever since they led the way, most other chain restaurants are now doing it as well. Some of the restaurants that offer low carb meals include: Applebee's, Arby's, Wendy's, Chi Chi's, and Boston Market

Dieting with low carb intake will help to boost your metabolism but only if you stick with it as a permanent lifestyle change. And that is the truth of it. It is simply safer that if you choose this method that you try to avoid taking any diet pills with it. All diets serve their purpose, but the low carb diet has been known to cause harm with certain people, so be sure to consult your doctor before committing to any of them.

The Benefits Of Alternative Methods

Alternative medicine can be a very difficult decision to make for most people. Visions of New Age robes and crystals can fill your head to the point where it just doesn't seem realistic when it comes to boosting your metabolism. Herbal remedies have been in the know for a long time. Many of the most well respected companies have moved into producing alternative products to meet the growing consumer demand for it. This is a blessing to most of the people who have chosen alternative medicine as a form of treatment.

It has been discovered and proven that prevention is the best medicine for most diseases. Taking regular doses of health supplements can stave off things like arthritis, skin blemishes and vision problems as well as loosing weight and boosting metabolism. Being mindful of good health measures is simple and well worth the effort. Believe it or not, Chiropractor's are considered as offering a form of alternative medicine.

Sometimes the benefits of alternative treatments are identical to those that are associated with more pharmaceutical varieties but the ingredients are what make all the difference. You do not want to introduce toxins into your system without understanding the negative effects. Not everything that can help you is actually good for you. Some good examples is in many of the diet supplements that are supposedly natural that can cause more damage than good.

Natural products are just as effective and potent as any others that are man made and in many cases they are better. They generally carry very high concentration of the desired substance and other vitamins and minerals as well. If you are ready to feel better and make a change, alternative medicine is your next best step to staying healthy.

Thanks to the constant demand for more natural products for boosting your metabolism, the FDA is now trying to control every herb in the world that has the potential to become popular. It is really bad that natural herbs are now becoming government property and by the time that you get it, many chemicals have been added to cause potential problems for you in the future if taken too long. If you really want natural, you should go directly to the herbs in their natural habitat. That is truly natural.

Alternative methods for boosting your metabolism are getting to be more and more popular every day. It is just a necessity of life. Some of the other alternative methods for doing this are to use hypnotism in order to change the way you function daily and your habits. It really makes sense when you think about it in terms of safety. If you are really looking to boost your metabolism naturally, diet and exercise help but if you lack the will power alternative methods can help change that.

<u>Breaking Through The Herbal Myth</u>

Herbal medicines and dietary supplements are not as strictly regulated to the arena of prescription drugs and over-the-counter medications, so it's important to trust the source before you start buying herbs as a means of boosting your metabolism. The most important thing that you need to know is what herbs are in the supplement or prescription that you buy. Since entire plants are often used in herbal medicines, consumers should be aware of the individual ingredients and the effects they can have on you with prolonged or short term use. A reputable dealer will always list the contents of herbal supplements for you or provide you with a pamphlet to explain it to you.

Because of the classification of dietary supplements by the Food and Drug Administration, herb manufacturers are not allowed to claim that herbs are effective for the treatment of diseases and other conditions but that is another story. But as history shows, herbs are time-tested throughout the world as a safe and effective way to battle certain diseases and afflictions.

Herbs act the same way as modern drugs and can be addictive at times, so it is important to use them correctly and not take more than the recommended dosage. Even though they are all-natural, taking too much of anything often can have serious health consequences. Some people also experience mild side effects from herbal medicines although most do not. That is why it is so important that you realize that even herbal drugs are still drugs.

While some doctors will prescribe herbal medicines as well as other treatments in combination, most people tend to use herbs without talking to their doctor. Because herbs contain many different compounds that may interact with other drugs like prescription drugs and cold remedies, people who plan to take herbal products should always consult their doctor before they begin. This is especially important for pregnant women, and people who take other medications and those who are especially sensitive to medications or certain herbal products. So before you start taking or buying herbal medicines over the counter, make sure that you know everything that there is to know first. It is just safer for you that way.

Just because herbs are natural doesn't mean that you can mistake this for being harmless. The same can be said of organic materials. Boosting your metabolism naturally doesn't mean that you can't get help it just means that you will not take any chemically based items to help you. There are many natural supplements that can help with your metabolism, but you still have to be wary. Do not take anything that without consulting a doctor. It is just common sense.

Combining Supplements, Diet And Exercise To Boost Metabolism

When we are young, our metabolism is naturally high, but as we get older that just isn't the case. Do you remember the days when you could eat anything that you wanted at any time and never seem to gain a pound? Those days were great, and long gone. However there is hope though. Of course we live in the age when we all want to find a quick and easy way out of everything. We want to find a magic pill that will change all of our lives, and the fact is there are thousands of them that claim to do just that.

Diet pills, which are also commonly called appetite suppressants, have been prescribed by doctors since the 1950s. When they were first introduced to the public, the majority of diet pills contained amphetamine which is otherwise known as speed. This drug is highly addictive and doctors quickly realized that appetite suppressants that contained it would not prove to be the remarkable weight loss solution they were searching for.

The big emphasis that just about every sensible weight reducing diet plan should be healthy weight loss, not fast weight loss because many of the 'fast' diet plans are not safe or healthy. With this in mind, the best type of weight loss is a calorie reduced version of a healthy balanced diet. This diet should encompass foods from all the various food groups that are outlined in any food pyramid only in good proportion.

Many doctors and physicians who research weight loss are now starting to focus on how low carb foods can help people trying to lose weight. The low carbohydrate foods that are currently available are unlike all healthy snacks that have come before them. They are tasty, and because of their popularity they are inexpensive and can make an immediate difference in how you look and feel.

When you try to boost your metabolism, there is so much that you can do without the use of drugs and other items. Just combining diet and exercise can do a great deal. All that is really needed if you want to is to use vitamin supplements. These are safe and they will help to boost your energy levels. You don't have to harm yourself in order to boost your metabolism, you just need to work at changing your lifestyle.

The Mediterranean Diet And Metabolism

Mediterranean diets are gaining in popularity because they offer low-fat, low carb alternatives to typical American diet foods. If you or a family member suffers from high cholesterol, you may want to steer your eating habits in a better direction. With great Turkish recipes and Greek recipes that are available online with this diet plan, it is easier than ever to sign up.

Also, Mediterranean diets are based on simple ingredients that are put together in a variety of delicious and exciting ways. Many people actually prefer to use extra virgin olive oil to spice up most of the dishes. The nutty, fruity flavor of the olive oil lends a delicious light touch to practically any dinner or lunch food. The good news for you is that Mediterranean diets depend a great deal on extra virgin olive oil.

The best part is that Mediterranean food is a snap to prepare. Making a Greek salad, for instance, requires only a few basic ingredients that you can purchase at any local supermarket. You can make your Greek salad with fresh lettuce, plump cherry tomatoes, wonderful kalamata olives, and a hint of balsamic vinaigrette topped off with feta cheese. Just the thought of such a salad makes most people want to head to the kitchen.

More and more, research is starting to point to the role of a person's diet in determining the likelihood of suffering heart disease. The best way to take care of your heart is to eat well before problems develop and not wait until the problem is there already to get started. That's why I encourage my family members and friends to eat lightly in the Mediterranean style. After all, too many fatty foods and thick, buttery sauces will clog your arteries and slow you down eventually.

The Mediterranean diet plan as well as others can be found online at ediets.com. These diet plans will help those who want to lose weight and those who just want to start eating better and healthier foods. Let's face it, 80% of the population in America is considered overweight and/or higher risk for weight related diseases. With those stats, can it be a wonder that so many diet plans are causing such a stir?

The Mediterranean diet is great for boosting your metabolism because it doesn't take away from your being able to eat what you like. The Mediterranean diet is popular because of the variety of foods that you can eat. It actually encourages you to eat often. Unlike the Atkins diet plan, this one does not want you to cut out anything and it really will help you to boost your metabolism without the use of drugs or chemicals. It certainly makes sense.

Using Food To Boost Your Metabolism

When most of us think about our metabolism it is mostly just in terms of losing weight. Our weight and our metabolism is what we use to define our bodies these days. The only problem with this is that we are also likely to forget that dieting does mean an absence of food, but the moderate intake of food. It is not healthy nor is it smart to take on all of those fad diets like the Atkins, South Beach or Zone diets that force you to completely give up certain foods because they only work for the length of the time that you are following that diet. If you do not continue that way all of the weight that you loose is only temporary.

Food is the key to boosting your metabolism and when it comes in its most natural forms, it can also be your best tool in maintaining a great weight for your body size and type. When I say natural forms I mean for example, when you eat vegetable and fruit it helps to eat them in the form that they naturally come in. if you eat fruit from a can, it is contained in syrup and sugars that will not be good for you so eating them raw is the best choice.

When you are eating vegetables it is best to eat them raw and steamed because it keeps all of the vitamins and minerals in them. You should also avoid processed foods and fried meats. Don't get me wrong fats are a necessary aspect of nutrition however saturated fats are not. The right balance of foods in a day can give your metabolism a boost that pills and fads can't.

<u>Using Natural Herbs To Boost Your Metabolism</u>

Herbal medicines and dietary supplements are not as strictly regulated to the arena of prescription drugs and over-the-counter medications, so it's important to trust the source before you start buying herbs as a means of boosting your metabolism. The most important thing that you need to know is what herbs are in the supplement or prescription that you buy. Since entire plants are often used in herbal medicines, consumers should be aware of the individual ingredients and the effects they can have on you with prolonged or short term use. A reputable dealer will always list the contents of herbal supplements for you or provide you with a pamphlet to explain it to you.

Because of the classification of dietary supplements by the Food and Drug Administration, herb manufacturers are not allowed to claim that herbs are effective for the treatment of diseases and other conditions but that is another story. But as history shows, herbs are time-tested throughout the world as a safe and effective way to battle certain diseases and afflictions.

Herbs act the same way as modern drugs and can be addictive at times, so it is important to use them correctly and not take more than the recommended dosage. Even though they are all-natural, taking too much of anything often can have serious health consequences. Some people also experience mild side effects from herbal medicines although most do not. That is why it is so important that you realize that even herbal drugs are still drugs

Dreamt Of A Great Body – You Can Have It

Ever had a dream about having the "Schwarzenegger" kind body? Well ,if that's true, then it doesn't have to be only a dream. Nowadays, fitness centers and gyms can give you the kind of body you dreamed of showing off. Know that body building is probably one of most sought after and popular sport in the States. Body building will give a muscular and built body one which you can flaunt when in the beach.

If at all you have extra flesh or those love handle's which you might find difficult to remove but no matter even how much exercise you do, you should really try working in a gym. Nowadays, Americans Body Building is giving loads of people who need to sport a perfectly thin, built and trim body. It's a proven fact that some extra portions of flab that you sport around can get really embarrassing, mainly when out near the beach side where you need to remove your shirt and try get a good tan.

Know that a good looking and fit body is always a very healthy body. Also know that working out using American Body Building, always be sure that the muscles will surely be toned and also your internal organs including the heart. Always know that it is not just the outside looks that counts but you need to possess good health if you want to fully enjoy life. And also, there is no point of a having a trim and great looking biceps, abs, tricep and all other muscles if in case you possess a bad conditioned heart.

Of late these supplements are now considered as the most popular and most publicized building product in the States. Most body building people from over the globe have given testifies that American Body Building supplements product offer very positive result in their main workouts and building activities and exercises. Now even the most world popular World Wrestling star John Cena is using American Body Building product. You might have seen how Cena looks like, then you get to know what you get by using those supplements.

There are loads of such products which American Body Building does offer. Most of their product is generally categorized into almost seven or eight kinds of supplement. It's more important that you are really serious regarding the workouts and also serious about getting the body you wanted in almost no time , and you must buy at most six or seven of their different products.

Ultimate Body-Building And Fitness

The main and first product of theirs is known as 'diet and energy'. This kind of product is generally used before starting the work out. But it will surely give you energy that you will need and also will nicely heat up the muscles to get it ready for some intensive working out.

The next product is known as the 'power and recovery'. Product is consumed orally only after a workout and it's mainly used for lean gain of mass . This tells that it will help the muscle to recover fast and also repair by themselves after the intensive working out to prepare for the next intensive working out .

In case you need fast delivery of the supplement, then you can try considering using some 'concentrated shots of American Body Building'. It gives you the extra boost of energy whenever you are doing a workout to complete the training in due time.

But after a workout, you can normally feel very dehydrated. Some of the ' the American Body Building pure hydration' products can help recover most of the essential fluid that might have been lost in the body.

After, before and during workouts, you might need some essential proteins in order to help the muscle to maintain its health and also at the very same time also develop. Some of the 'the American Body Building hi-protein' will help get the muscles to be trim all the time.

In case you decide to enter body building competition, then should try some of the 'hardcore essentials' products offered also by the American Body Building. But this is so packed with all the supplements and its also tested in order to get the great body and same time also give best result in trimmed and lean muscles.

So incase, you are searching for the way to a muscular body which you can happily flaunt, then you must consider doing the working out to the extreme possible with some American Body Building supplement.

<u>Body Building Diet</u>

When one thinks of body building, one must not limit their horizons to extensive work out and exercise alone. Diet, one of the most basal components, should not be ignored at any cost as it complements the process to achieve optimum potential. Apart from providing the daily need for calories it supplements the body with the essential nutrients and vitamins.

Carbohydrates predicated to be an indispensable part of the diet, especially for body builders are found abundant in breads, pastas, beans, potatoes, bran, rice and cereals. Carbohydrates contain 4kilocalories per gram and are the storehouse of energy for the body. Hence complex carbohydrates via starches and fiber are a big yes.

Next comes Protein which is vital for building tissues and muscles in the human body. Physical activity and exertion as well as enhanced muscular mass increase your need for protein. Proteins like carbohydrates contain 4 kilocalories per gram. Proteins can be obtained from varied sources which include meats, eggs, grains, legumes, and dairy products such as milk and cheese. Body builders may require up to almost one and half gram of protein per day, say like 6 kilocalories.

The general misconception people have is that Fat is bad. They fail to realize is that there are different categories of fat, some of which is necessary for the proper functioning of the body. The functions of fat include- fat in the body is converted to glucose to release energy, serve as a buffer against diseases and also promote healthy cell functioning.

Thereby making the right choices like unsaturated fats(olive oil, flaxseed oil, etc) over saturated fats(cocoa butter, palm oil, etc) can play a major role. One must be aware that saturated fats lead to diseases like the coronary heart disease. For the layman, one can distinguish physically between the two, by noticing that unsaturated fat is found in liquid state and saturated fats in solid state at room temperature.

One must also take in large amount of vegetables and fruits as a part of their diet for body building. Various vitamins and nutrients which are mandatory for the proper functioning of the body are found in vegetables. On the other hand sugars and roughage are aplenty in fruits. They also play a role in retaining water.

Ultimate Body-Building And Fitness

Finally adequate roughage or fiber in the diet contributes in many ways like providing satiety in the diet, improving bowel movement and is a good source of vitamins and minerals. Apart from that it helps reduce weight too. Avoid peeling off the skin of fruits and vegetables, eating lot of green leafy vegetables are good sources of dietary fiber.

A exemplary body building diet incorporates all the components and ensures it is balanced and high in nutrients. One must make sure that there are about five to six small meals dispersed through the day instead of three big ones which large intakes of protein and carbohydrates in the morning. One must never skip the breakfast ,the most essential meal of the day. When one knows the key for body building is good diet, nothing must stop you from going for it!

Body Building National Championship

There are many choices when you plan to compete in a body building contest. The choices are diverse in a body building championship in the national level. There is not just one national champion in body building. It is just the weight category that makes a person more famous than the others.

Various establishments come forward to sponsor the body builders in a national level championship in body building. NPC national level championship in Body Building is one of the best contests when it comes to serious body building. The National Physique Committee is the most respected establishment of the lot and all their national events are attended by many body builders for the award.

Most of the championships are actually sanctioned by the National Physique Committee. Just the NPC brand is more than enough for people to enter the competition take part in it by carrying some weight. For all you might know, if you win, you will hit the hall of fame and carrying the title around with a pride that only a few people have had!

The Amateur Athletic Union is yet another establishment that is a major sponsor for these championships. These are more for the amateur people and rookie body builders. This is like the stepping stone for more serious competitions in their lives.

The contests for Ms. and Mr. Olympia are also considered as competitions for national level championships in body building. This was actually made a household name ever since Arnold won this title back in the 70s.

There are national level championships held by some magazines based on body building and fitness. Viz. Muscle and Fitness, and Flex are magazines that sponsor the contests and the winners of these editions are featured in their magazine. These are seen as a great opportunity for a person who is looking forward to serious body building.

It is always better to compete in national level body building championships when it is being sponsored by famous organizations like National Physique Committee. You should always be in

Ultimate Body-Building And Fitness

top form when you are competing in national level championships because the others there are looking forward to the same fame that you are trying to achieve.

If you are talented enough to be victorious in a national level body building championship, then, you will be a prized body builder. It is something that you can always be proud of. It is only after you win a national level body building championship that you will be considered good body builder.

So, keep the vision alive, go there and participate and give others a hard time. It cannot be accomplished in a night; it is a penance will surely reap rich dividends.

Body Building Supplement Review-Eat Right To Feel Tight

Body Building is a sport which requires more than just the spirit to build your body. Consumption of supplements will help you get a new shape all together. There are loads of supplements that you can choose to actually build your body.

The supplements can be used as per the ideas that you have to build your body. It is the choice of the right supplement that will make the difference. The most appropriate one will help your workout. Here is a review about the legal and popular supplements that are used to build the body.

Creatine

Creatine is used in many areas in body building. This is the supplement used to add on the muscle mass and help the body builders gain more strength. Creatine is also used to kill the fatigue in the body builders after their heavy workouts. It enhances the body metabolism and processes food in a better manner and reduces the cholesterol in the system.

Nitric Oxide

Nitric oxide is used to enhance the performance of the muscle building agents in our body. It also helps you to increase the weight you lift, and it boosts the output, apart from these, it quickens the process of muscle contraction. In addition, it is believed that nitric oxide enhances the stamina and their sexual feelings.

Proteins

Protein is given primary spot in any body builder's diet. This acts as the building block in muscle building nutrients and it helps build mass in all possible ways. This is an amino acid which helps in building really well toned muscles that are fit. Carbohydrates are the best form to take the protein supplements. The Whey Protein is one of the quality protein supplements that any body builder uses to build his muscles the way he wants.

Glutamine

Glutamine is often referred to as 'sexy sister' of creatine. Coincidentally, glutamine is an amino acid produced by the body naturally. It is to be noted that the level of natural glutamine found in our body decreases due to the stress on the body, including the workout stress. The absence of glutamine would tarnish all the hard work that you did at the gym, as it leads to muscle loss.

The fitness magazines make it a habit to actually review all the supplements that are used in body building. The reviews always help the body builders by letting them choose what they want, based on the type of body they want. Just reach out for them and tone your muscles up.

Body Building Workout

A workout followed by any body builder must be a properly planned program that gives enough attention to all the areas in the body and enough resistance to all muscle groups. It should contain all forms of exercises like cardiovascular rotation and weight training. There are various types of workouts for building your body.

The current position of your health matters a lot for devising a proper workout for building your body. Your body condition influences your susceptibility to an injury, and your recoverability from any other injuries. There is a certain limit up to which the body can take the workouts. It is always suggested to slowly increase your level of workout, start slow and keep reaching higher regions.

The personal goal is another factor that matters a lot when you begin to workout. It is always better to get your preferences right by deciding if you want an increase in the body mass, or lose weight or become stronger. If the workout is done depending on the goal, the chances to succeed are much higher.

Having a basic knowledge about the location of muscles is very important when you decided to workout. The basic idea about the location of the muscles will help you flex them to the maximum possible extent.

Regular body building workouts are generally done up to four days a week to start off with. The best days to workout are Monday, Tuesday, Thursday and Friday. Take off on Wednesday and weekends. Below is a good workout chart that will help you focus on all parts of the body:

* Day 1: Triceps, Deltoids
* Day 2: Traps, Back
* Day 3: -Rest-
* Day 4: Forearms, Legs
* Day 5: Biceps, Chest
* Day 6: -Rest-
* Day 7: -Rest-

Ultimate Body-Building And Fitness

This kind of a workout will make you stretch only one part of the body and it will give maximum recovery time for all the parts which gives a maximum potential for growth. It is important to give the correct recovery time due to the heavy workout, and it will heal your muscles between the workout sessions.

The progress needs to be kept note of regularly and all the exercises must be noted. This will give you a basic idea as to where you stand when you consider the strength potential. Changes can be made in these workouts to realize any personal goal of yours.

The workouts done to build your body vary with each person. But the basic workouts remain the same and it helps all body builders tone their muscles the way they want. Put the entire workout together to keep your body strong and fit.

Body Building Supplements For Females

A sport that is rapidly gaining popularity in our advanced society is female body building. It is now widely accepted that women with a toned physique are regarded to very sexy and sought after by men of every kind. That is the reason for this steady increase in interest in women for body building, which was once considered to be a guy thing.

If you are the kind of woman who wants to improve her physique then enrollment in a gym and a body building course is almost mandatory and much better solution compared to crash diets and other harmful exercise patterns. Since the body of a man is very different from that of a woman, the methods and program for building the body for woman are different. Even internal workings related to various chemical and hormonal changes are very different for men and women

The knowledge of the nature of supplements to be used constitutes the first part of the program. Care also has to be taken to retain the feminine form, otherwise one could end up looking largely built and manly.

Such programs for women are generally less though than what men undergo as it is a biological fact that the female form is more fragile than the male form and hence extra care has to be taken. Supplements specially made keeping the female form in mind are also available nowadays. Creatine monohydrate is one the newer supplement to hit the markets. Sometimes this is also used for men but specially made Creatine monohydrate for women are also available.

Liver, kidney and the pancreas generally produce these variants of supplements. Creatine monohydrate is also known to be useful in tissue damage repairs in muscles and also for extended endurance by many athletes who are generally more prone to such muscle and tissue damage than the other people. Keep in mind that muscles in the body can be damaged to due building the body and at times these damages can be very harmful and cannot be reversed. Use of Creatine monohydrate supplements will enhance the muscle healing and reduces healing time and thereby the muscles which undergo stress will be back in form in very les time.

Good news about Creatine monohydrate is that it is perfectly legal, one hundred percent. Assuming this substance was not allowed, consuming meat products, which also have a huge

content of this compound, will not be allowed also. Consumption of this is very essential for the body and hence is very safe and needed.

Some multi vitamins specially made for women also help in muscle repair and building. In addition few proteins are also specially made for accumulation of body mass for women.. Keep in mind that proteins are the main reason for muscle tissues. High protein food will also help the accumulation of protein in the body. But proteins got from food is very less. Hence whey proteins are used for the better absorption of protein to the body.

All the above mentioned are the best supplements available for females now consultation and advice of a fitness trainer about eating these supplements is very important because it takes more time for the female body to prepare itself for the high intensive workout . Remember that only hard work will get you that perfect physique in spite of all the
Supplements.

Take care to keep all these things in mind about the supplements for body building. To get that perfect body you have always dreamed of, make sure you use proper supplements with instructions from your trainers.

Discount Body Building Supplements

The best deals for body building supplements can be struck at websites online. They give the best discounts. None of the stores will give you jaw breaking discounts on the supplements used for body building as the ones you find online do. It is because of one simple reason; they buy it all in bulk and they dispatch it worldwide to the people who are interested in buying them from you and passing on the money online.

There are more than a million websites ready to sell you supplements for a discounted rate. We will list the top sites for you now.

* **www.evitamin.com** – This website is a good find, that not only gives discount price on supplements, but also on vitamins. They carry almost all the brands that you can possibly name, and sell stuff at half the retail price.

* **www.worldclassnutrition.com** – Name the supplement, you will get it here; there are millions of good quality, branded body building supplements available here. This site is extremely trusted for its loyalty towards its customers.

* **www.supplementstogo.com** – It is very good website that sells all the supplements from different brands and also sells vitamins. They give detailed articles about the different supplements for the customers to be informed.

* **www.bodybuilding4u.com** – This website gives a thorough review about the different supplements apart from giving the best advice on where people can find discounted supplements. They give good tips on body building and exercises for specific parts.

It is really important to do your own research on a supplement before you buy it, even if it is a company product, with a good background. There are several unscrupulous sellers who might try to sell the wrong supplements and promise to you that you will get the desired effects. And these supplements might not help, and might have a side effect on you.

Trust and follow brands, it is very important when it comes to selecting your supplements. It is because it might go a waste in case the supplement does not give you the desired effect. If you manage to convince your seller to give you the discount price on the brand that you specify, then, you are the winner.

It is essential to find a particular place where there is a review for specific supplements used in body building and then find a place where you can get them at a discounted price

Female Body Building Videos- Strength Knows No Gender

The female body building's popularity is soaring to levels unseen till date. This has lead to a point where there are many videos showcasing this sport. Women are obsessed with their bodies nowadays, so they are looking forward to build a great structure and showcase the same using videos.

Women who are seriously into body building are suggested to make their own videos. Most of them own video cameras. Just take the help of a friend, and try posing in different positions and then workout all the parts in your body to make sure they are at the maximum potential.

It is not a disgrace to be checking the female body building videos, in fact, they are a source of inspiration to keep your body fit, seeing those women work their body out to perfection, you are inspired to do so, and it helps a lot. There are a lot of libraries where the female body building videos can be found.

There are many websites hosting the body building videos. There are a lot of options for you to select from, women posing for competitions, performing exercises, etc. These videos can very well be your motivating factors to keep your body fit.

The hardcore websites dedicated to body building will surely host a series of women body builders' videos. Apart from this, they offer a lot of variety and we can see some of the top women working out.

In case you are not a member of any gym, make sure you become a member in some local gym, and take their advice when it comes to shaping your body. They will be able to give you precise information about the best female body building videos that can help you in a longer run. They can give you a few places where you can find these videos. Many of the local gyms have their own collection of gym videos, which might include videos of body building by female. These videos are a food for your interest in body building and a guide to accomplish a goal of getting an enviable shape.

Ultimate Body-Building And Fitness

Do not spend a lot of money on these body building videos, just check the internet for the videos, you are sure to stumble upon many. Viewing those videos will surely help you reach your goal in body building.

It is a misconception that body building is a sport taken up by men, women are also taking equal interest in this sport off late. When you come across the body building videos with women, just take a note of what these women do to keep their body so beautiful. Take advice from them to make sure your body looks the way you want it to be!

Insulin In Body Building

Insulin is a normal hormone which is secreted by pancreas in reason to very high sugar level. The main use of this is regulating body sugar levels. The utilization of insulin for body building is a very controversial topic as utilizing it equated as using steroids and its also used to better a workout.

When the sugar levels in blood are high, this tends to hike the storage of the glucose which mainly gives energy to the whole body. Benefit of this for body building is that it provides more energy and allows longer and even tougher workout. While this insulin does create an anabolic environment within the body, but it can only cause more harm than any good.

All diabetics cannot produce their own supply of insulin and that is why they take synthetic insulin or get a control in their insulin production via diets. In case you are not diabetic, consuming insulin when not needed will cause the pancreas to halt production naturally. And what is the result of that in the end? It will essentially make you a diabetic.

But unfortunately, for the body building universe, this is readily got incase you ask for it. This is like a shot once in a day and also is often utilized to be "bulked up" prior to body building competition if any by the hardcore body builder.

This will tend to "force feed" the muscle with lots of sugar. Hike in sugar will let longer workouts before exhausting you, it will cause danger to the normal insulin making ability.

No way are we endorsing use of any of the artificial substance in body building programs. Always strive for a healthier body before you start workout. Taking substance like this into the body amounts to your body not being in good condition.

But for a diabetic person, insulin is needed. It kind of saves their life and helps them live a normal life with diabetics. When this is utilized in body building, it leads serious complications that affect the ability to continue in the sport which you most probably love. Don't take ant chance with your health – irrespective of your goals .

Ultimate Body-Building And Fitness

Use of insulin in building can cause serious health injuries even coma, and increased pressure, and also a hike in the respiratory rate. Don't risk health and well-being.

<u>Natural Body Building</u>

In a sport like body building, there will be many supplements that are used to grow the muscles very quickly, but most of these are man-made steroids substances. The natural body building done is without the use of unnatural materials being put inside the body. But that does not mean that not using supplements as many like the available natural products. What that means is that staying away from such man developed hormones and steroids in order to help building the body mass.

Body building industries have taken a firm stance on use of the illegal and artificial materials - mainly competitions. There even are some specific contests geared for the natural body builder. Most of the competitions will test them before allowing them to contest, and if they are found to possess an illegal material in the body, they will be banned from taking part.

While all the synthetic products will enhance the body quickly, they might have bad side effects. Trend about natural building is all about growing the body and maximizing nutritional intake and as well as stay healthy while growing the muscles.

After you have decided that natural building is how you want to do it, then it's important you take the correct amount of all the vitamins and nutrients that will enhance your workouts. This means popping a multi vitamin and also eating properly will send all the muscle building protein to the correct parts of the body.

It's definitely possible to enhance the body naturally by way of an effective training program along with decent nutrition. There is absolutely no reason for steroids or growth hormones to be put into your body for building some muscle mass.

The key component of the natural building program is to make sure you eat healthy and also keep a positive mindset about the workouts. Sometimes supplements are important if you want fit, toned muscles. The key ingredients in such supplements like glutamine and creatine are produced in the body anyhow. What these supplements do is hike up substances that are present there anyway.

Ultimate Body-Building And Fitness

All Proponents in favor of natural body building will surely agree that effective workouts along with good supplements and proper nutrition will make for a fit, healthy and toned body. Natural building is surely the way to do it if the goal in the bodybuilding program is to feel healthy and good. Some steroids and some growth hormones must not be used at all.

Building the body the natural way is perfect for all. Steroids surely are not. so don't take that chance and suffer bad effects after steroid use. Keep in mind that a good workout program and commitment to the body building goal will surely grow the body in the natural way not otherwise.

Natural Body Building Supplements: The Way To A Healthy And Fit Body

Natural building supplements provide various advantages. All these supplements are food extracts which contain nutritional dosages made in such forms that are easy for body absorption. Normally, these are not other means for basic diet but additions along with normal diets.

Natural body supplement can help get the proteins, vitamins and minerals you need. Intake of such supplements depends on the purpose. But it does not need a large dosage if you just want an athletic and fit body. Very small dosages of the minerals and vitamins are sufficient. Incase you want to have rippling muscles, then go for liberal dosage of these natural building supplements, especially protein supplements.

In any case, enthusiasts have to learn to make the most of it. In case you want to consume any natural building supplement that reveals your need to achieve fitness and other health objectives. Do keep in thought that these supplements have to be accompanied by useful activities. In order to keep fit and healthy, you require the force of the mind and body and the spirit. Any simple natural building supplements wont do any magic .

In order to maintain a healthy lifestyle, proper diet and exercise is needed. All natural body building supplements only aid the body to do its activities naturally. Generally exercise never means getting fat or thin. It only promotes healthy brain functioning and healthy blood circulations. You can feel relaxed, stay organized, gives you needed energy, and also sleep better in the nights. If only you pull together exercise and the natural supplements, that way much better results are got.

There are many natural building supplements in the markets today. They also promise to hike your performance and also health status. In case you enjoy any fitness activity, you can get benefits from all these supplements. Do not just take a chance. Always do research to know the genuine supplements. All manufacturers give their best in order to convince people to buy their product. And as much possible, go through unbiased reviews about the effectiveness of the supplement based on sound analysis. Quick results for getting the lean muscles then use the

Ultimate Body-Building And Fitness

better building supplements. Know that, the better natural building supplements works effectively and also does no harm.

Looking for the better supplement must be done with logic and intelligence. In case you are careless about the selection, then there is a risk of having a harmful side effect and also losing money . Also try to avoid doing untested experiments on the body and try to do cardiovascular exercises.

Take advice from many experts like a professional gym instructor. It helps you to create a idea how all these supplements boost a persons fitness desires. It is needed to realize what kind of natural supplement you can take, in respect to the vitamins and nutrients that are suitable for you. That will enable to get enhanced muscle growth.

And finally, you need to understand fully the mind's capability. Remember that bad emotional and bad mental states can also makes person unwell. To get the correct value of these natural supplements, make sure your attitude stays positive, also take enough rest, and make sure to keep the mind free of stress. Doing all this with natural supplements can guarantee a healthier, happier life.

The Bodybuilding Supplement – Nitric Oxide

Chemical compound symbol for the Nitric Oxide is NO, it's a gas essential for signaling the molecules. In specific, it correctly controls blood circulation and also regulates the function of the brain, stomach, lungs and liver. In addition, it's responsible for controlling the blood pressure. Specific to men, it helps in dilation of blood vessels for penile erection to happen.

It's said that NO is a highly helpful body building material. Building supplements are responsible for all the muscle build-up and also getting rid of unwanted fat.

Heightened flow of blood is the most needed aspect of NO and that's why it's very important to many bodybuilders. They are generally benefited by the some of the following:

- Nitric Oxide also improves the blood flow and makes way for the nutrients to be correctly delivered to all the muscles. And as an end result, there is perfect growth of muscle during the adaptation and also during the recovery stages.
- Nitric Oxide also reduces inflammation present in the body. Hence, the muscles are protected from great stress.

Other health benefits of NO also includes:

-Protects the individual from the chances of heart problems since it helps in protecting the blood vessels.
- It also aids in the prefect control of platelet functionality.
- It is known to reduce artery plaque.
- It also helps to lower cholesterol levels.

There are many different kinds of NO supplement present in the markets.

1. The MRI NO2

These kinds of NO supplements are noted to be an important find in bodybuilding supplements. The MRI NO2 creates a continuous muscle pump.

2. The BSN Nitrix

It's not a hormonal supplement and does not cause hormonal imbalance. The primary function of this is to boost NO levels in your body so that an increased blood flow can be got.

Three of the necessary nutrients which are there and which can be found in BSN Nitrix are L-Citrulline, Phosphoplex, and Nicotinamide Adenine Dinucleotide called NAD.

3. The Pinnacle NoX2

The most important ingredient of the A-AKG and the A-KIC is to make the product efficient in order to lengthen the muscle pumps, and also enlarge and rejuvenate muscles.

It's said that the Pinnacle NoX2 is same as the MRI NO2. But the difference is about the cost of products. The latter is much more costly.

4. The Syntrax Nitrous

These kinds of Nitric Oxide body building supplements are a kind of powder supplements that makes them easy for digestion. Arginine ingredient is mixed with the malic acid hence makes Syntrax Nitrous very effective for the correct secretion of insulin in the body, production of the energy and muscle recovery.

The utilization of such samples of NO body building supplements must first be talked about with the trainer. Need for the supplement can vary from person to person. There are side effects that can be neutralized with use of products having NO like:

- High Nitrous Oxide dosage can cause vomiting and diarrhea.
- Also cause frequent headaches.

Apart from NO supplement, you can get the natural sources with food having L-arginine like meats, milk products, fish and grains.

Ultimate Body-Building And Fitness

Uses of certain body building supplements have it's own distinct advantages and also disadvantages. In order to get optimum results it is recommended you take the supplements in the recommended dosage.

Bodybuilder's body will not be got by taking supplements alone, you also need to do tough training, and be careful with the diet and also get enough rest.

Body Building: For Teenagers

Teenagers can benefit from bodybuilding in a number of ways. Bodybuilding is of course a great way of keeping in shape and maintaining good health. However bodybuilding can allow you far greater rewards than a mere good body. Read on to know more.

A number of parents are concerned about the kind of effects severe exercises (such as those necessary for bodybuilding) can bring about to a teenager's body. A teenager's body, as we all know, undergo a number of natural changes. Hence, parents are concerned that the additional strain of heavy exercises might prove detrimental to the teenager's growth. While there is no real proof to suggest that exercising can harm bodily growth most gym instructors are of the opinion that teenage bodybuilder's often suffer from a particular problem that has much to do with their being a teenager. This problem concerns the usual impulsiveness related to being a teenager. Teenagers enjoy breaking rules and disobeying instructions, while this might be a fun thing to do usually in the gym while working with weights nothing could be more harmful than being a rebel. Bodybuilding is all about discipline, and teenagers do not, as a rule, like discipline. This is the sole problem that plagues all teenage bodybuilders.

Many people believe that working with heavyweights can stop bones from growing. They justify their claim by pointing out that lifting heavy weights can quicken the closure of growth plates, thereby stopping their growth far before they are supposed to. While this logic sounds watertight it is yet to be proven as true. Also, groups opposing this theory have pointed out that most professional athletes (many of whom had begun training with heavyweights at a young age) have not strictly adhered to this rule and remained stunted. Thus, as of now, there seems to be no solid proof to suggest whether or not weights affect a certain individual's growth.

Even if working out with particularly heavy weights does actually have an affect on the bones of teenagers even then none of them are really in much danger. This is because such an effect can really be harmful only before a teenager reaches a certain level of maturity, and majority of teenagers reach the full extent of their growth by over and around the age of 15. Now, surely no 13 or 14 year old will be pumping iron to build his body and thereby getting his bones all arrested!

Apart from the growth issue there is the issue, which we already discussed and which concerns the basic problem of being a 'teenager'. Most teenagers feel out of place being neither adults nor children, as a result they try to hasten their life and 'grow up' quicker than they are likely to naturally. This 'quickening' causes many of them to try and emulate everything from the walk to the talk and even the workout regimes of their seniors. Obviously this can prove a disaster since teenagers are not technically supposed to do things that an adult does. An adult bodybuilder has far more stamina and experience than a regular teenager, as a result emulating him can prove taxing and even dangerous for a young teenager.

To ensure that they don't end up hurting themselves real bad by trying and imitating better trained adults all teenage bodybuilders should preferably hire a trainer for themselves.

Body Building: Software

All bodybuilders wish to have a powerful physique. That is why they are bodybuilders in the first place. Body building software can be a huge advantage to bodybuilders because it provides them with technical information on how to train, what to eat, and when to rest for maximum recovery in order to get the maximum benefit out of each and every workout session and meal.

If you believe that body building is nothing more than weight training and cardiovascular exercises combined with well planned high nutrition meals then you are mistaken. There is a whole lot more to bodybuilding than simply that. You also need to know how to train, how much to train, when to train, and when to give yourself a timeout. The same applies to all that you eat.

It is not enough to simply go by what seems right. Body building software is like a personal trainer that can keep on the straight line to maximum growth and strength.

Besides being educational body building software also has the added benefit of accurately keeping track of all your activities and your growth and performance. You may use the software to plan and record your day to day routines, calculate the calories you used in your workout and how many you are going to take in your meals. All this makes it easier to know where you are going on a daily basis.

The best way to look at body building software is in the sense of a partner that is constantly giving feedback on your performance and indicating areas where you need to work harder. It will help you fine tune you entire routine to get the most out of everything you do for your body.

Body building software is quite affordable so there is no need to worry about the cost. There are many software available that can suit any budget. As with any other software the cost of the one you buy will depend on the features built in. Just shop around and you are sure to find one that covers everything you need and also fits in your budget.

Some of the best body building software are actually written and even include videos of well known fitness trainers and expert body builders. These also include useful information for all bodybuilders. The software includes a questionnaire that covers things like age, gender, fitness level and so on in order to create a customized fitness plan for anyone using the software.

Ultimate Body-Building And Fitness

There is also body building software that comes with prediction capabilities that help you visualize the sort of results you may expect by following specific routines for specified periods of time.

Body building is as much an art as it is a science. There are technical and skill based factors that determine the outcome of everything you do in the gym or at home.

Body building software is simply a tool that helps you to do everything right while keeping track of your accomplishments and suggesting areas of improvement.

Body Building: The Basics

Though bodybuilding appears to be a modern day activity it has its ancient roots dug deep into 12th Century India, where the very first training methods and bodybuilding related diets first emerged. Within 300 years bodybuilding had become a phenomenal success in India and people from all over the world were following their lead. To assist their bodybuilding attempts people created their very first dumbbells and weights during this time. With the creation of the first weights weightlifting and bodybuilding found its foremost element.

In the western world bodybuilding came to be recognized as a great sport only in the 1800's when bodybuilders such as Eugene Sandow came to the forefront. By the early 1900's people felt a growing need for the introduction of contests that would validate the hard work of those who built their body. As a result, the bodybuilding competitions, which have become such a quintessential part of the whole regime today, came into being. Sandow was one of the frontrunners of the initial bodybuilding movements and was named the father of Modern Bodybuilding. To make sure his voice and ideas about bodybuilding found its way to the people he made frequent public appearances, organized exhibitions and, more importantly, started the pioneering fitness magazine 'Physical Culture'.

It was Sandow who finally pushed the authorities of the Olympic Games to include weightlifting as one of the events. Thanks to his efforts weightlifting came to become one of the main attractions of the Olympic Games from the year 1896. Even today it is one of the most viewed events of the games.

With the arrival of bodybuilders such as Charles Atlas in the bodybuilding circuit in the early 1900's the sport became even more widespread and lucrative. Quickly his legendary ads spread all over the place and penetrated deep the deepest psyche of all American men. Everyone in the world wanted to be just like him!

Quickly more and more exercise equipments started gaining popularity in the market. People were now getting conscious of the way they ought to train, the way they ought to eat and the equipments they ought to purchase in order to sculpt their body into shape. The fitness industry was only now shaping into the form we are acquainted with presently.

Ultimate Body-Building And Fitness

With the emergence of the Tarzan and the Hercules movies between the 50's and the 70's bodybuilding became something of a rage. Everyone was now raring to go and achieve a body as beautiful as Steve Reeves.

Cashing in on the cult status of bodybuilding was entrepreneurs such as Joe Gold (who found both, the Gold's Gym as well as the World Gym) and others.

Bodybuilding was now struggling to segregate itself from weightlifting and become a sport by itself. During the 70's yet another bodybuilding phenomenon by the name of Arnold Schwarzenegger was to take the world by a storm with his perfectly carved body. Later he would enter the Guinness Book of World Records as the best developed man in the world and thereby begin a cult of sorts.

Body Building: Safety Measures

Bodybuilding requires hard work and tremendous discipline. To build your body you will have to work extensively with heavyweights and irons, to ensure that neither of these have a detrimental effect on your muscles or injure you in anyway you will have to take a few safety precautions. Start by reading up a lot of material on careful bodybuilding practices like those that instruct you about appropriate weight lifting methods and ways to warm up and cool down etc. In the next section we will discuss a few essential techniques you must exercise at the gym.

Always begin with a proper warm up and end with a warm down session. Each should take no less than 15 minutes. Take 5 minutes to jog and at least 10 minutes to stretch your muscles and prepare them for what's coming and only then plunge into the exercise regime. Remember to go from low to high. Start with the lighter weights and slowly go up to the really heavy weights. Let your muscles get accustomed to the idea of lifting weights and prepare themselves to use up the body's strength.

Identify exactly how far you can go. No one except you yourself can decide how far you ought to go, since only you know what your limits are. Its good to challenge your limits but don't overdo it and end up straining yourself, even the best of bodybuilders can cause terrible damage to their body when they are strained.

Remember, bodybuilding might involve evaluations at contests but the process itself is not a competition so you don't have to prove yourself to anyone. Take your own sweet time to prepare yourself to take on heavier weights. In case you feel like you are overexerting yourself, simply ease up and take hold of a lighter weight. Definition and muscle amplification is a result of calculated restrain and not uncalculated risks such as those involved in lifting excessively heavyweights.

Get yourself a spotter to watch your moves when you are working with particularly heavy weights. Your spotter should preferably be of your own strength and someone who can help you out with a tough spot in case he/she finds you submerged in a troublesome situation. To ensure that they are loyal to the cause however make sure you act as their spotter as well. Most bodybuilders ask their training partners to spot for them. Spotters are essential for getting you out of a particularly tough weight situation. A number of people hurt themselves while working

with weights. If unfortunately you too experience such an accident your spotter will help you out, contact the gym staff and take you to the hospital if required. Even if you do not get caught in such a soup your spotter will help you stay motivated and keep you focused on your immediate goals. You can return him/her the favor by doing the same for him/her.

As soon as you get a basic idea of your training program and know the exact forms you should take in order to ensure that the program proves beneficial for you start working in front of the mirror to see if you are staying true to the forms you have been advised to take.

A number of people hurt themselves simply by assuming the wrong positions while training. Watching yourself on the mirror ought to keep you from making such mistakes.

Body Building: Exercises

Perhaps the most simple and efficient exercise to build the body, not necessitating starting gear, is the leg squat. Later weights used across the shoulders and hands can also lead to considerable muscle increase.

And still, it can be one of the most effective exercises you can use to maintain muscle tone and build definition in pretty well all of your leg muscles.

The leg squat is so simple and easy an exercise to perform that it can be done while being engaged in some other activity. So even while attending phone calls or while cooking, you can keep one eye at the stove and also do the leg squat. Of course, it's important to be careful.

So multitasking isn't a problem with quite a few exercises

For the leg squat, comfort is a priority, and not feeling well or being up to it can be quite dangerous. Doing it incompletely or doing it poorly can be even more damaging than not doing it at all.

This is how you prepare yourself for the leg squats:
1) Firstly you must stand with your legs placed apart. The most convenient width between the two legs would be shoulder width. Loosen your body y giving yourself a little shake.

2) A succession of deep breaths should follow, and the breathing should ensue from the stomach rather than the chest.

3) It is important to relax. Concentrate on your body and try to gauge how able your body is to take the exercise.

4) Gradually lower your body while beginning the leg squat. Bend gently down at the knees. When you go down do remember to exhale.

5) Stop and hold on for a few seconds at the lowest point. This is most important in the whole of the exercise. Inhale when you raise your body.

Ultimate Body-Building And Fitness

This is an easy exercise but immensely beneficial. You will find your muscles tightening over a period of time.

The number of reps is up to you. Don't start big initially as that can prove to be damaging. As you increase you'll gain strength and vice versa. You can slowly increase the number as you progress, and you will realize that it is not as simple and more taxing than you at first believed.

Beginning with leg squats is very good for the legs. After a bit you can use small weights and even advanced working out simply means progressing to larger weights across the shoulders.

It basically implies working out the muscles in the leg. Selecting a few muscle groups to add more pressure on to also means adding variety.

For instance, standing with toes directed slightly outwards would work on the muscles of the inner thigh.

On the other hand, if the toes point inwards the reverse happens and the outer thigh gets worked on.

Leg squats as the foundation of your bodybuilding routine will definitely take care of your legs. However it is important to take ones time and gradually build up the reps and the weights.

Body Building: Diets

If you want to flaunt a great physique and body and have started working out, then you must realize that a good diet also helps you go a long way.

The diet is often ignored during the course of a bodybuilding program. While the imperative is working out, diet is no less significant. It helps to make the muscle mass leaner, and your body fitter. It maintains energy levels and loses the flab.

A bodybuilding diet program is all about knowing what foods you might consume and how you can take care of the various nutrients that you require by incorporating them in your diet plan.

If your eating routine is not healthy enough then it is time to bring about a few necessary changes. This is vital for a healthy and fruitful lifestyle, a disease free life, and a healthy body.

The following are some pointers that can assure you of the success that you desire, provided you follow them:

1. Carbohydrates are a must. It is required to develop the muscles that store glycogen. It also helps to maximize athletic prowess.

Carbohydrates must be eaten in their minimally processed form. For instance, whole wheat should always be preferred over white bread. Carbohydrate should contribute to approximately 50-60% of your total calorie intake. This depends on the workout as well.

These are some of the foods, which are full of carbohydrates and recommended as part of your diet - wild rice, squash, oatmeal, baked potato, pumpkin, whole wheat bread, brown rice, or a sweet potato.

2. Protein is also an essential constituent of the diet, and also very important for an athlete in the process of bodybuilding.

Next to water protein is the most plentiful substance found in the body. It is found throughout the human body - muscles, skin, bone, and the blood too. If you are training and building on body

strength, then protein is required to build muscle mass.

Of the total calorie intake 15-20% should be protein. Protein rich foods that may be recommended during strength training are turkey, salmon, lean ground beef, low fat cottage cheese, egg whites, chicken breast, and sirloin steak.

3. Water is vital for workouts. Drink plenty of water. It is indispensable in sustaining the performance level of the workouts. For intensive routines a glass of water (8 oz) is a must every 15 to 25 minutes.

This is again necessary to maintain the metabolic rates and strike a balance between the various nutrients. It will help to burn off calories faster and more efficiently.

However it is important to consult a physician before venturing into a diet or rigorous exercise. Healthy eating and bodybuilding are synonymous.

Body Building: Supplements

When it comes to bodybuilding supplements, what can help you immensely is the ability to come to a decision.

Muscle building can be brought about effectually and in a natural way by supplements such as vitamins and minerals. The market has also seen a rise in the use of artificial supplements. These are known to have potentially damaging effects but bodybuilders choose them for their capacity to produce a spectacular result in a short period of time.

One of the leading contenders in the bodybuilding supplement market is called Cell-Tech. This supplement, once added to your protein shake, enhances creatine in the body. This is an ideal supplement to be used after an arduous workout since it serves to replace the burnt out cell mass.

The sugar used up during the workout is also replenished by Cell-Tech. There is an immediate surge of insulin in the body on the ingestion of Cell-Tech that prevents you from feeling the after effects of fatigue after the workout, allowing you to continue with your normal day to day activities.

However, a salient point that is to be made is that the key factor in the bodybuilding routine is not an external supplement but internal motivation. If you are determined to build your muscle mass and lift weights regularly in a disciplined schedule then it would be as effective as consuming steroids.

Weightlifting, being a natural method of bodybuilding, is probably better. After consultation with a physician it is not even potentially dangerous. Another fact that you must keep in mind is to add a certain degree of variety to the routine. Otherwise, the muscles adjust themselves according to the exercises and do not develop.

Other than weightlifting other excellent supplements that may be used are vitamins and minerals. A multi-vitamin pill taken daily can help your body to absorb more vitamins and minerals in general.

Ultimate Body-Building And Fitness

It is good to make certain that your consumption of good fats is in the right proportion. Good fats and flax oil are present in foods like peanut butter. These are necessary for muscle building, though only if taken moderately.

All these techniques and pointers are useful but what is of paramount importance is the need to follow a strict diet chart. A plan of nutrition and food must be made. Also avoid large meals and invest in several small ones as that helps your metabolism to increase and burns fat.

For maximum benefit to body it is wise to consider integrating calorific cycles into your routine. If you want to lose weight then you could have high calorific intake for three days and low for two. An appropriate bodybuilding diet would have the right proportion of these constituents i.e., carbohydrates (40%), proteins (40%), and fats (20%).

The best bodybuilding supplement is thus generated within the body itself. Muscle cells undergo division and multiplication in this unique natural process. Vitamins and foods loaded with minerals is the healthy approach to bodybuilding.

Thus, traditional weightlifting and exercise scores above synthetic supplements in many respects.

Body Building: Equipment

Body building truly became a craze from 1970, mostly due to the movie Pumping Iron featuring, no prizes for guessing, Arnold Schwarzenegger. While trying body building, it's important that you consider your goals first. Is it to build muscle mass, to lose weight or to tone up?

The equipment you choose to use whether at home or gym, depends upon these factors. The most basic need served by body building, as the name suggests, is to develop muscles mass. For this you need a pair of free weights which, apart from being the most effective body building equipment, are also the least expensive. Add to this the fact that they are portable, come in a variety of designs and you know why they sell like hot cakes. Free weights are the most useful fitness equipment as they can be adapted to your workout by increasing the weight as you get used to your current program.

Body building is also a sport now and for those interested in training for the profession, a proper routine in consultation with a specialist and a doctor would be advisable. As far as the fitness regimen goes, a weight bench with a set of barbells from ten to forty pounds is ideal for building large muscles. Just work your way up gradually to the heavier weights.

For those who don't want the definition of the professionals, dumbbells are the way to go. Easy and portable, one can even get a pair of aquatic dumbbells to practice in the pool. This is especially for those with back problems and arthritis. Pull- up bars and push up stands are great for toning your upper body and arm sculpting, as they take it through all its paces. Focus on frequent but less number of reps for toning and intense reps twice or thrice a week if you want bulk. Dip stands on the other hand, give your wrist that extra support and help in strengthening your arms and hands.

Whether a professional or otherwise, keep in mind that you need to alternate and supplement your exercise routine with the adequate nutrition and rest. Body building is tremendously taxing and you need to take care if you don't want to end up hurting yourself. Even though you might want to work out everyday, remember that your body needs to recuperate between workouts.

Depending on your fitness level, aim for one to five serious workouts per week and gradually increase the intensity and duration of your workouts.

Ultimate Body-Building And Fitness

Finally, be patient. If you have never exercised in your life till date, chances are you will take some time getting used to it. Make a routine, consult a doctor and a specialist, get proper nutrition and stick to your regimen. Your efforts will be rewarded in due time.

Body Building: The Art

There are various kinds of bodybuilding but at the basic level all of them involve growing muscle hypertrophy to the greatest extent possible by means of a proper diet, regular rest and proper weight training. Bodybuilding is considered by many as a means of beautifying the body, in much the same way as a temple is beautified with carvings. But while many engage in body building simply due to the fun involved in it many others are into competitive bodybuilding and regularly participate in body building contests where their physique and appearance is judged by a series of judges.

Bodybuilding at a competitive level often involves obtaining, developing and preserving a well-worked out, aesthetically pleasing body and balanced physique. All competitive bodybuilders work towards certain standards set in the circuit and thereby try and prepare themselves according to what judges at a contest might expect them to be like.

Competitive bodybuilding lays a lot of emphasis on posing in various ways so as to show off every muscle in the body. Body builders practice all the poses they assume during the shows while preparing themselves.

Right posture, posing and of course the right amount of development of the muscles is what earns favor with the judges at these contests.

A body builder need not be particularly strong! It's true, despite being expected to be engaged in rigorous weight training bodybuilders are not ultimately judged according to their strength but rather according to the shape and size of their body.

All those who engage in bodybuilding, even at an amateur level know how taxing it is. Bodybuilders all over the world not only have a stringent exercise regime, but also a rigorous diet. Above all however it is the level of their discipline which helps them clinch matters and earn a body worth showing off in a contest.

Bodybuilding is nothing like sports such as weight or power lifting because, as we mentioned previously, it lays less emphasis on the strength of the muscles acquired and more on how aesthetically pleasing the muscles and the whole form of the body is. Thus either sport is based

Ultimate Body-Building And Fitness

on totally different fundamental principles and can therefore hardly be compared.

Bodybuilding is of various types. There is of course female bodybuilding, which has gained popularity with time, then there is teenage body building, natural body building and of course the regular professional bodybuilding.

Professional bodybuilding is all about participating (and then winning) competitions authorized by the IFBB. Only if the builder manages to go through with the qualifying rounds of these at an amateur level and thereby earn a 'professional card' can he/she hope to participate in contests of the kind. Once they win these contests the builder will be given a chance to participate in the Mr. Olympia contests, which is deemed to be the greatest title in this field.

The popularity of teenage and female bodybuilding is a recent factor and shows how popular the sport has become with both teenagers as well as women. Teenage bodybuilding is really a stepping-stone for future bodybuilders, most of who begin on their quest to bodybuilding fame and fortune during their teenage years.

Body Building: For Women

For the longest time female bodybuilding enthusiasts were cowed down by the cry that 'women do not belong to bodybuilding' and 'it's a man's sport'. Even women themselves were of the opinion that bodybuilding was not particularly 'feminine' since weights and muscles supposedly didn't 'look good' on women. It took a long time for this attitude to change and for women in the field to be finally taken seriously.

Today, however a large number of women have managed to successfully break out of this stereotype and taken up bodybuilding and fitness training at a professional level. A variety of women take part in the regular bodybuilding competitions happening all over the country, all of them look 'feminine', fit, beautiful and stunning all at once.

Women who want to take up bodybuilding often hesitate about looking 'manly', but they couldn't be further from the truth. A great physique is not necessarily a masculine trait. A number of female bodybuilders are downright beautiful women, in the conventional sense and their built up body has just added to their glamour, not taken anything away. If you exercise consciously and with a well-defined goal you to can preserve you womanly softness despite having developed a bulky body. In fact the entire notion of looking 'manly' when gaining muscles is absurd since men and women are structurally different and no woman, no matter how much bulk she manages to add in terms of muscles can possibly look like a man!

This is because men in general have a different stature than women and women almost never become as big as a man regardless of how muscular they may become. Contrary to popular belief bodybuilding has often been known to make women feel more 'feminine', a large number of men too find such women particularly attractive. But that apart, bodybuilding is known to augment one's level of confidence to a large extent.

Women who engage in bodybuilding claim to feel 'more confident' and 'in control', a feeling that slowly permeates through every aspect of their life.

It doesn't matter what your particular body type is, you can be slight or big boned, tall or tiny but you'd still be able to reap benefits of bodybuilding. This is because bodybuilding is not the same thing for everyone and different bodies can be built up in different manner. For instance if you

Ultimate Body-Building And Fitness

are slight begin with small weights instead of heavyweights, which can be harmful for you. However if you are slightly broader and stronger use medium sized weights, which will be far better for you than the small weights used by small framed people.

No matter what your final objective is chances are you'll find a great little niche within the bodybuilding circle for yourself. The bodybuilding circle has been known to accommodate everyone from the chance amateurs, who is seeking nothing more than a well toned body to a really serious professional who is primarily interested in winning all contests. Gone are the days when female bodybuilders were considered to be shiny young things clad in skimpy little bikinis and therefore ogled at mindlessly. Today female bodybuilding has earned itself the sort of respect every sport desires to.